White Fir

Essential oil

Clearing Karmic & Generational Patterns

By: Stasia Bliss

This book may be shared in part or in its entirety by any means. You don't need permission from the author, for you and the author are ONE in the Divine Human Family. Use discretion and kindness.

First Printing: February 2015

This book and all the books in this series are dedicated to the ever renewed birthing of the Divine Self – for which the gifts of essential oils are continually given.

Table of Contents:

Caution - - Disclaimer - - Personal Health Observation -

This book is not a replacement for therapy, medicines, or treatments of any kind. It is merely meant to give a new perspective on the uses of the essential oil mentioned herein.

It is advised that through realizing yourself to be the only One you can change, that when things seem bleak or undesirable, when health or life seems to oppose you, that you instead choose to seek to affect change within yourself rather than look outward for "cures." This book in no way intends to heal or cure you or act as a replacement for medical or psychological treatment, it does intend to lift and inspire you into your own greatness and sovereignty. Proceed at your own risk and free-agency.

"A man doesn't plant a tree for himself. He plants it for posterity."

— Alexander Smith

Introduction

" The meaning of life is not to be discovered only after

death in some hidden, mysterious realm; on the contrary, it can be

found by eating the succulent fruit of the Tree of Life and by living

in the here and now as fully and creatively as we can.

~ Paul Kurtz

This book continues on in our series about Essential oils for Consciousness. In the previous book, we discovered the healing power of Arborvitae, the great western cedar and explored the virtues of that sacred tree which many call "the tree of life." As the quote above urges, after we have eaten of that tree, partaken of the fruit as such, we must find a way to live in the here and now as fully and creatively as possible. This next book in the series is perched on assisting us to do just that.

White Fir is yet another great and mighty tree which holds many secrets and mysteries for the uncovering. In this book we will learn how, by utilizing white fir essential oil, we may slough off the energetic blocks which hold us back from living fully and completely in the here and now.

White fir is a powerful oil to use following the use of Arborvitae and they complement each other in their application. For as Arborvitae helps one to find roots, get comfortable and ecstatic in the suit of embodiment we wear and further the path, White fir continues the journey by bringing to light those things we no longer need and helps us to let them go.

There is no coincidence that the great trees step in to assist us first in this journey of realizing deeper consciousness through essential oils. They have been standing through time and dimensions to watch and wait for this opportunity to share the wisdom and the gifts they hold for us.

Let us step now into the arms of the magnificent White Fir and learn of her treasures.

In the Family —

"You can't heal the personality or relationships of one child without healing the whole family. The influence of the family tree is too strong. If you had the opportunity to explore transgenerational behavior patterns, as family therapists do, you might be surprised at how easy it is to predict that a particular personality trait will repeat itself in a specific child in the family sequence. Most people have "psychic octopuses" that need to be cleared out of their personalities. Tentacles originating several generations back can still jerk you around like a puppet on a string.

Because we are so intertwined with our ancestors, we can't lift ourselves out of our harmful patterns without lifting our entire family tree out with us." (Denny Ray Johnson, What The Eye Reveals, Rayid Publications, 1995, p75)

A large grouping of trees is a forest. A large grouping of people is a family, one that extends far and wide and deep. The trees which grow tall together lend stabilizing essences that can help to ground us and put our feet firmly on the floor, rooting us into our nature.

Trees like the arborvitae, spruce, pine and fir all like to be around each other and support the grouping principle. In many ways, this is beneficial to them as species and to those animals and other creatures which seek refuge within their care.

Likewise, families become places to seek shelter within, to be supported inside of and sometimes to hide in. Often, when feeling alone or weak in the world, people will retreat to the home of their blood family, or to the home of those who feel like family.

Family creates solace and space for meditation upon our possibilities as well as engenders a sense of belonging and provides hope for a future to develop and thrive.

Within the forest, trees grow together and ensure their longevity by standing strong side by side. They provide a constant and necessary cloud of oxygen to our earth and the inhabitants thereof and provide recreation and beauty to all.

There are many glorious and positive qualities about families and forests, the grouping of life and the sharing of resources. However, there are some aspects to grouping and family that can be negative to the individual – whether tree or person. Let us look at what these aspects are and how we can navigate them and potentially remove those that are possible to leave behind while maintaining the grace and blessings from interconnectedness.

Family, by its very nature, shares and passes along things: ideas, beliefs, patterns, belongings, stories, love. Some of these things benefit the progeny and some do not.

Genetic coding can actually record beliefs and patterning, behaviors as well as emotions and pass them on through DNA to a new human without explanation or choice.

"A particular pattern will continue to run in a family until the pattern is broken or resolved. Unfinished business from an ancestor can affect our lives and actually show up in the DNA and the eyes."

- (see What the Eyes Reveal, Denny Johnson).

What we have received from our family, our parents, grandparents and long into the past, is not always known to us and can influence the way we live, make decisions and can contribute to blocking attitudes and behaviors which keep us from living our greatest potential.

As trees, who drop their cones and create offspring near to them, watching them grow to stay solid in the earth and populate the forest which makes up who they are together, like the old saying goes, an apple doesn't fall far from the tree.

If a tree tries to grow too close to its parent tree or trees it might become stifled by their branches or even stunted in growth.

We become who we come from because we carry the imprints within us to do so. Some of those imprints are beneficial and positive, others – not so much.

The great news is we can utilize essential oils, like White fir, to help us to release those patterns, beliefs and behaviors which are not ours to carry and free ourselves to have a life that is uniquely ours.

"Our genes determine much more than our physical traits. They influence how we think, feel and react, shaping the course of our health, wealth, and relationships. Emotions affect and alter our DNA- and, conversely, our DNA affects our emotions, attitudes, and behaviors. The emotions that impact our genes come not just from experiences we had in this life. We inherit the emotional patterns and beliefs (or "stories") of our ancestors. Deeply imbedded in our DNA, these ancestral stories influence is in ways we are not even aware of. We are not prisoners of our genetic heritage. Our genetic codes are flexible, not fixed. Through simple, but powerful self-healing techniques, we can reset our genetic codes and with them the stories of our lives." (Margaret Ruby, The DNA of Healing p 19)

Get the Point –

It's in the Needles

White Fir essential oil is distilled from the needles of the tree, which seems very significant to the topic. Ancient health traditions such as Ayurveda and Chinese medicine have identified the body as being covered with acupressure points and meridians, or lines of energy. In an otherwise healthy, open and connected person, all the energy centers and meridians (or nadis) would be open and flowing fluidly.

When there is "stuck" energy or blocks in a person, these blocks manifest as a pain in the body or a tension in the field, which can show up as a "negative" emotion or other unhelpful feeling or experience.

I like to imagine that our entire body, upon development, was imprinted with all that energy and understanding that came before us, as if the needles of a White Fir tree were pressing down into our skin – in all the acupressure points.

Some of these energies worked for us and they still do. We, in many ways, may be like those who came before us – our parents or grandparents – and are here to carry on the mission they set out to accomplish, just at a higher octave of manifestation perhaps. So, these "points" work for us and do not create blocks or stuck energy.

On the other hand, other imprints have pressed down heavily on our energy body and seemed to have punctured the fabric of our lives. Energy seems to leak out through these areas and patterns have been created in our lives – mentally, emotionally, physically – to deal with and compensate for the impressions we were unconsciously bestowed.

White fir is a great gift for releasing these impressions, especially if we become aware of what these imprints are first.

It is not necessary, entirely, to know what is being released in order for White fir essential oil to assist, but it is good to be aware of the process and tune in as much as possible.

White fir essential oil seems to trigger the points which have stored the stuck energy to purge and release. These stuck patterns can be from before you were even born, given you through your DNA and manifested in your field as they were for those who came before you.

You may not even know what it would be like to live without the patterning that you have been existing within. White Fir is a gift for the unveiling.

Applying White Fir externally to the skin while imagining it seeping into each and every acu-point or choosing specific points to apply it to can increase and speed up the rate at which white fir may help you release old patterning.

From the oil of the needles to the points on the skin, white fir essential oil is meant to work with the process of peeling the layers, triggering the points and enabling the true you to shine through.

Dots, Patterns & Karma

"The second chakra deals with karmic patterns. As you awaken and clear this center it can often trigger what some term a 'dark night of the soul'- for within this center lays all the muck of lifetimes past which must be overcome and transcended in order to evolve."

~ Stasia Bliss

In Eastern philosophy there is this concept of karma, that what you do creates something for you later – either positive or negative. It is not too unlike the idea of cause and effect. Though karma, as it is believed in and taught in the east, is thought to extend beyond the grave into multiple lifetimes.

In some ways, generational patterning and karmic debts are not too dissimilar. Something is being passed along from the previous owner, whether it is directly you – in a previous life – or your predecessors – the results seem to be pretty much the same. A pattern is created, a belief is stored, and it is played out without choice by the carrier.

In the yogic tradition the chakra system is recognized as playing a crucial role in the evolution of consciousness. Each chakra corresponds to a level of awareness and as the centers are opened, purified and activated, the awareness and perception is likewise cleared and transformed.

Where one would view life from fear of survival and safety, when functioning with a dirty or closed first chakra, for example, an open and cleansed first chakra would allow one to know that all is provided by the universe and there is plenty for everyone.

There are various stages and levels for clearing out and it is not to say that someone worrying about survival issues has a totally blocked first chakra and is stuck there, for there are layers and stages to the cleansing of all the centers. But this is the basic principle.

When dealing with karmic issues and generational patterning, the second chakra is said to be responsible for the storing of this information. What is interesting about this is that the second chakra is also responsible for procreation, general satisfaction and joy.

One who has not dealt with generational clearing and the release of patterns from the past is stuck in a pool of muck where joy and satisfaction cannot be fully realized. The second chakra is associated with the water element and one literally is swimming in muck before the clearing of this center.

Another key to the water element ruling this center is that water represents emotions. The emotional body is where we store generational patterns, they are like stuck emotions. As we identify these and release them, a flood of cleansing energy rushes over us and through us to allow the pristine pools of joy to fill.

White fir oil assists with the clearing of this vital center as well as helping clear away the blocked emotions as they surface for release.

Sometimes, when we are in the midst of noticing our stuck emotions surfacing, simply applying White Fir oil is enough on its own. This powerful oil can sweep the energy field clean and allow for dramatic shifts in the body and emotions.

Other times we need to implement additional tools to assist in such profound and great work as the removal of old, stuck patterns sometimes stretching back hundreds of years and dozens of generations behind us.

This next chapter briefly highlights a fantastic supporting tool for use with White Fir essential oil.

Releasing the Sap —

Emotion Code

"Trapped emotions and messages are stored over our lifetimes, and perhaps transmitted to us from our ancestor's lifetimes through the DNA."

- (Quantum Healing by Deepak Chopra.)

We often need a bit of assistance in identifying the sappy intruders in our beautiful temple embodiments. I have recently happened upon one of the simplest and most powerful tools to assist in this process and I have found that it works absolutely amazingly with White fir essential oil in releasing old, stuck patterns in the body.

This system was developed by a Dr. Bradley Nelson and is called *The Emotion Code*. After having worked for 25 years as a chiropractor and implementing muscle testing in order to tap the body's innate intelligence to find out what was really going on, he found that nearly 90 percent of issues afflicting people today have to do with blocked emotions.

As I have trained with Dr. Nelson and used the Emotion Code on myself I have found so many things changing in me. I feel lighter, clearer and life seems to have become simpler and more streamlined. White Fir just kind of jumped on board with me during this process and proved itself invaluable in the mix.

Every time an old emotion was released using the Emotion Code, I would literally feel that emotion like an energy climbing out of me or off of me and sometimes it would hover, or stay stuck-ish on the surface. With that I would apply White Fir essential oil and it would act and does act like a peeler, removing those emotions and energies which have surfaced much in the way a snake skin would be peeled off. That is my experience.

The Emotion Code, as referenced in the back, is a simple method you can use on yourself by asking your body to reveal what emotions you have been carrying around through muscle testing. You can also visit a practitioner, such as myself, or have a phone proxy session with outstanding results.

Many times, stuck emotions identified through this method are found to be inherited. When this is the case, White Fir is particularly called for. But in all cases, the oil is soothing and assists in the transition from that old released pattern.

For more information see references in the back of the book. Know that no matter if you use the *Emotion*

Code or not, White Fir, on its own, is an excellent tool for helping to sweep away old stuck energies and patterns. *The Emotion Code* only makes it that much more effective and fast.

Shedding the Layers

Patterns, beliefs, stuck emotions, inherited or self-made, all these things we carry around in layers. We have been acquiring them all of our lives only to realize now that we are too thick for our own good. We have protected ourselves from our own essence, our power and our truth.

The time has come for the walls to come down, the patterns to become organized and healing, and the truths to be known. We have lived under the illusion that life had to be and continue as it was, full of dysfunctions and obstacles, for too long. It is time to shed the layers and discover the pearls which lie within.

White Fir essential oil is a gift to those who wish to transform and peel away the layers which no longer serve. It can be used to assist in breaking habits, releasing negative thoughts toward things, letting go of addictive behavior and changing a routine that seems no longer helpful or positive.

It is easy to get stuck in ruts even if they were not our idea in the first place. Sometimes we find ourselves repeating language or thinking thoughts that someone else told us or we heard say often. These became programs we are running and we do not have to continue running them.

The same goes for pain. The body often times creates pains and aches in order to get us to listen to it. Once we do, once we start to pay attention to what our body wants from us it can start to release the help cries.

By applying White Fir oil to areas which ache or feel tension, we are, in effect, telling that part of the body, that tension, that we no longer need to keep the negative emotion that was attached to it – that we are listening and can therefore release the block.

If the body is acting out with pain, some stuck emotion or pattern, White Fir oil will change the energetic vibrational frequency of that area to not match any longer that of pain and discomfort. It will receive the new frequency.

Do not be discouraged if things do not shift entirely all at once. Remember, we are layered like an onion. We have compounded belief over belief over pattern over emotion and it must be taken down and peeled off.

Never ignore acute, painful, warning-like symptoms. Always take care to see a professional if it is warranted. You will know when that is. Using essential oils is a more moderate approach to symptoms and situations that are handle-able by you.

Remember, however, that you are stronger than you sometimes give yourself credit for. Be willing to feel some discomfort in your body as you shed old beliefs and patterns. Recognize the difference between psychological pains and acute physical ones.

White Fir oil is a gift in helping to remove old layers of you that no longer serve the you that is ever unfolding and developing moment by moment, day by day. This process of becoming is on-going. White Fir can become a generous companion as you travel the trails of unfolding on this journey of life and awakening.

Once you release many generational blocks and purify the emotional body, you will begin to see more clearly... as if you are staring through a crystal clear pool. Things will slow down in your vision so you can catch them and remain unsurprised. Things become more fluid, more beautiful.

Before this happens, when you are peering through murky water, life feels a bit scary, uncertain and cloudy. Clearing the generational patterns and the karmic ties passed down from your family line and through the DNA is huge on this path of evolution. It changes the game entirely.

As you peel the layers, always remember to affirm that you are in fact peeling them. You are not the you that started this whole thing. Allow for a change in perspective as you say goodbye to the you that used to be. That skin is peeling. That you is dying.

This death is a renewal, a new birth.

As we peel away the old and release the stuck emotions, we are truly allowing our lights to shine. We are forgiving the past for ourselves and our children. We are opening hearts and healing the world. So much new can be created when we are through dealing with the old, out-dated. These are exciting times.

White Fir has been waiting a long time to share this with us. She is so thrilled to be here to serve in this capacity. The conversation between White Fir and our bodies has been initiated. We may continue this dialogue as we progress through the healing and release of generational and karmic patterns. By discovering and acknowledging emotional blocks and using essential oils to intend release, we are telling our DNA that we no longer wish to be carriers of lifetimes of dysfunctional feelings. We are speaking a new language to ourselves and to our children, that of healing and fluidity and power.

"You may not think that you can 'talk' to your DNA, (another prejudice that comes from seeing DNA as only a material blueprint), but in fact you do continually . . . . Thinking happens at the level of DNA..." (Deepak Chopra, Quantum Healing, Bantam Books, 1989, p 234)

Best White Fir Applications

Topically – as needed

If you have sensitive skin you can dilute in coconut oil or other base oil. You just may need a drop or two of this generous and abundant oil. It seems to go a long way, just a little bit. Rub over areas of tension or pain. Imagine the pain/tension leaving the body, peeling off like a snakeskin.

Breathe it in –

Diffusing this tree oil into the atmosphere can assist in lightening the mood and calling out the inner you to surface from behind blocking emotions or patterns. The scent is an invitation to step with trust into a new life, one that is full and rich and majestic like the forests.

Take note that diffusing White Fir can break up habits and patterns in an area too. When this happens it can sometimes be akin to things flying up in the air and spinning around before they fall to reveal their next best place or space. So, unless you want to rearrange or feel new somewhere in your home, just take caution in stirring the atmosphere up with this gift of change and release.

By that same token, White Fir can help break up congestion in all its many forms – resulting in "breathing deeper."

Over the navel/2nd Chakra –

To assist in the activation and purification of the second chakra/energy center you can apply White Fir right to the lower abdomen and/or several centimeters up from the base of the spine. When doing so, imagine clearing the waters of this center and breathing in the visual of pure, pristine fluid there

Souls of the Feet – applied to the feet, this oil can assist one in grounding to the Earth and feeling the supportive energies available to all from the core of the great Mama. If one is feeling stuck, unable to move, White Fir can help mobilize one into action by assisting one in noticing the opportunities presenting themselves in day-to-day life.

Top of the Head – applied to the crown, White fir can connect one to the remembrance of a time and space more Divine and pure. It has the potential to decongest our memories as to who we really are and where we came from. It may relieve mental or emotional pressures and the tendency to dwell on the inharmonious or incongruent. The third eye can be gently stimulated into action for assistance in continued healing and release during dream-states. Using *The Emotion Code* work with

White Fir almost always results in clearer dreaming and vivid recall. This oil is ideal for meditation and harmonizing both hemispheres of the brain, supporting Alpha rhythms and peace.

Heart – Over the heart center, White Fir helps to support the gentle opening of a closed heart, especially when the heart has been blocked with generational or inherited patterns of fear. After removing a heartwall with The Emotion Code, White fir is idea for placing over the heart center and high heart to facilitate greater connection to the self and to others emotionally. It can support one in realizing and remembering unconditional love and the ability to self-heal by tuning one into the inherent energies of wholeness within.

Divine Child of the Universe, anoint thyself with oils for thine own remembrance, for Ye are Gods!

Resources:

The Emotion Code: www.healerlibrary.com

doTERRA essential oils – www.doterrauniversity.com

To buy this oil visit –www.mydoterra.com/blissinthehouse

My personal website: www.blissinthehouse.com

43